Welcome- *Thank you for purchasing this book. The information in this book I have researched, studied and put it to the test. I took it upon myself to learn Nature's Techniques to self-healing. Using food, fresh juice, air, water, exercise, Turkish towel rubs, meditations and visualization.*
I am not a physician, I do not claim to be.
I am relaying my story to you through experiences and research of my own learning.

Na-is-Tru-to- Al- *is an acronym for*
Nature is True to All *(A Kwini Souleimane Production)*

Be True to Your Nature and Nature will True to You
(Tanya Childs-Souleimane)

The Creator works through the Creation *(Tanya Childs-Souleimane)*

Time to Start Living and Stop Dying

Dedicated to the Divine Creator of the Universe and Emmy Ross, who was right by my side at the beginning of this journey.

What Prompted this Change?

In 1995 my body went through a complete physical breakdown. I was highly over weight and had developed tumors in my arms and legs. I became very ill to the point of death. Weeks prior to my physical breakdown I was led by divine intervention to a health store, there I purchased a book entitled "Back to Eden." I learned and studied the techniques, applied them and healed myself.   In 1998 I re-infected myself again this time using myself as a guinea pig. I began to take notations on the effects that processed foods had on the body. In doing this my research became more profound.

In conclusion I have come to find there is No-Way around Nature's food. The fruit of the tree is for man's food and the leaves for his medicine. (Ezekiel 47:12)

Born with a Survival Kit It's wonderful to know we
have a great creator to watch over each and every living being in the universe. Knowing that, wouldn't you think the Creator had enough sense to put us here with a SURVIVAL KIT! Everything we needed for our survival was created at the beginning of creation. The Creator never needed any help from man to make anything extra to feed his creation and to top it off- harm his creation. "HMMM"
So a plan was put in place for the day awaiting our mess-up.   The plan was always in the most popular book in the world for those who say they believe in it. But I'm finding this very hard to believe being people don't follow half of what is written. Now don't get me wrong, some things written in the book is confusing and hard to understand. This is when you need to know someone who can decode the book. Let's take a look inside the most popular book written. The Bible.

Look at 1 Timothy 4:1-5 this is taken out of context. Somewhere between these verses people got confused. The verse does not mean YOU CAN EAT ANYTHING- PRAY OVER IT AND YOU WILL BE ALL RIGHT! No- if that was true, why are you still sick with high blood pressure, diabetes, heart disease, kidney problems, highly overweight, aches and pains and whatever else is ailing your body? WHY? You think God really told you it was alright to pray over your food than you eat it and it makes you sick. That would mean God is deceiving. God is not deceiving- Man is. The point is you can't pray over dead food and think you are going to be alright. Dead food is anything processed, anything that has been stripped of its natural state and someone has added extra artificial additives to make you want it more- as well as causing health problems in the end. These foods are known as taste good foods. Someone is saying I like taste good foods.

Be aware Taste Good Foods are Acididocis –meaning these foods turn into acid in your body. Therefore an over accumulation of acid in the body turns to disease. Cancer, Tumors in body, High Blood Pressure, Diabetes Heart disease, all kinds of aches and pains in joints which is arthritis or rheumatism skin problems and more.

NITRATES/NITRITES (According to Ruth Winter author of Fifth Edition a Consumer Dictionary of Food Additives)

> Nitrates/Nitrites both are Potassium and Sodium mixture.
> Potassium nitrates also known as saltpeter and niter used as a color fixative in cured meats. Both nitrates are used in matches and to improve burning properties in tobacco. They combine with natural stomach saliva and food substances (secondary amines) to create powerful cancer-causing agents. (*Ruth Winter, M.S*)
> Note: In all Meats- except free ranged meats

<u>**Yellow 5**</u> is Tartrazine- derived form coal tar and Salicylates- is salts of salicylic acids – to much of this taken in could cause stomach pain, skin rashes, vomiting, *and mental disturbances.*

<u>**Red#40**</u>

Is Erythrosine which is a coal tar derivative, a brown powder that becomes red in solutions? Causes cancer in animals, and skin rashes and hives. This red dye cause *hyperactivity and psychotic behavior* in people and the children are full of it.

According to Ruth Winter author of Fifth Edition a Consumer Dictionary of Food Additives

N- CARBAMOYL ARSANILIC ACID- White, nearly odorless powder added to animal feed as a growth stimulant. It is arsenic. On the Community Right to Know List. Poison by ingestion. Has caused tumors in lab animals. *(Ruth Winter, M.S)*

Now let's fry it- Flour has been bleached using Calcium Sulfate or some other bleaching agent. Then add the Partially Hydrogenated Oils to cook it in. The chicken is no longer chicken, it has become a purely poison by ingestion, therefore over consumption of this item lead catastrophe on contact.

Solution- Free range chicken- boil and baked.

Go to your foreign markets to get it.

You have to have patience here. If you fry the chicken it has to be cooked in an oil that is from a pure source.

If you don't want to do this – limit your intake tremendously

Hydrogenated Oils

Wow- This mess is definitely in 90% of what we eat especially fried chicken and other fried or baked food products.

What is it anyway? Glad you asked – (*According to Ruth Winter author of Fifth Edition a Consumer Dictionary of Food Additives)* Oils that is partially converted from naturally polyunsaturated fats to saturate. Makes liquids oil partially solid. May adversely affect (meaning harmful) the levels of fat in the blood and has been linked to colon cancer in some reports. *(Ruth Winter, M.S).*

MSG- is in almost every processed food we ingest
According to Ruth Winter author of Fifth Edition a Consumer Dictionary of Food Additives
MSG-Mono-Sodium Glutamate.
Accent-Zest. The monosodium salt of glutamic acid. Causes brain damage effects in rats, rabbits, chicks, and monkeys. Depression, irritability and other mood changes have been reported. Reproductive Dysfunctions, fewer pregnancies, reduced fertility in males. Results on animals in labs. Headaches, chest pain and numbness reported from china diners. *(Ruth Winter, M.S.)*

These are only a few additives, my point is, you can't pray over this stuff and think you are going to be alright- it just doesn't work that way.

The passages is referring to natural food of the earth that is from the land without being tampered with. And if you are going to eat flesh meaning animal flesh it has to be free range and all the blood must be drained from it. A note to the reader (Flesh was only eaten on rare occasions not every day and certainly not in the way we are eating it today.) Please note meat is not flesh as we know it today- meat is the fruit of the tree. We are calling the wrong thing meat, we got it all twisted up. (Flesh is Flesh and Meat pertaining to Fruit which is the original name for meat, not animal meat- that is Flesh) sounds ick when you think about it – Huh!

Now let's take a look at the clues it leaves about how to eat, actually the book is loaded with it.

Ok, I'm not preaching I'm teaching now. So don't get it twisted. Psalms 103 v 5. Who satisfies thy mouth with good things; so that thy youth is renewed like the eagles "fit's me perfectly, YEAAA!" Look at Genesis 1:29 God gives herb and fruit for meat. Genesis 9: 3 and 4 every living thing shall be meat for you, even as the green herb have I given you all things. *Every living thing shall be meat for you-*

*l*ook at this closely and open your mind- YOU CAN'T EAT A LIVING ANIMAL- you have to kill it first. So living prefers to vegetables and fruits, the fruits and vegetables are living the only way they become dead is when you cook them to death, I hope you know what that means. You know when the greens are cooked for 2 hours and have no more color in them and when the fruit is limp and has no-more crunch or firmness to it. Hope you are getting this. Look at Numbers 11 v. 33-34 In short when we started eating flesh (meat) we came down with plagues of the body. Meaning diseases of today.

Here comes Isaiah 40 v. 6-8 it tells us all flesh is grass and all the goodness thereof the flower of the field. Ok don't trip here – pay attention you have to look at Genesis 2:7 where it tells us we are made from the dust of the earth.

The trees and plants comes from the earth, so that means plants have the same elements our body needs to function. The plants have basic elements *carbon, oxygen, nitrogen,* and *phosphorus,* these elements makes the grass grow and live, our bodies need the same basic elements *oxygen, carbon, hydrogen, nitrogen, calcium,* and *phosphorus.* Both have the basic elements to survive. Everything lives and thrives on vegetation. So, why not leave all the unnecessary junk and go straight to the source.

Now, I'm not trying to make you a vegan or vegetarian, just note that flesh meat is not to be eaten daily it was only used on special occasions and it had to be prepared correctly. Simple if you're eating flesh meat- eat free range and make sure the blood is drained out of it and don't eat it every day.

On the last note look at Daniel 1:8 and 11-20. Daniel fasted on vegetables and water and was able to see clearly of his surroundings. He gained knowledge, wisdom, and visions more than all the others in the kingdom. I can testify to this.

Now, I really like this example, King Nebuchadnezzar was made to eat grass for 7 years- after during this, his understanding returned to him. Some research shows the cells in the body replaced themselves in 7 years, some believe some don't. Fact is I transformed my body in 5 1/2 years. So whether it's 5 years or 7 years. It can be done!

How I did it

After being led by divine intervention to a health food store where I purchase the book and learned the techniques along with helpful information from other sources, I comprised everything together and went to work on myself.

First, let me tell you my warning signs. My flesh felt like something was crawling on me, I would itch all over, then I would feel sharp pains, like needles were poking in my body. I would get nausea at times. My skin turned a grayish ash color and I was real cold, you could feel the lumps in my arms and legs and on the inside of my hand on the thumb area. I would go numb often all over my body. I remember having to walk for weeks in my small apartment and not sleeping just to keep my blood circulating to stay alive. Later my flesh began to detach from my bones-you could put your finger in my flesh and it would leave a dent. I was sick, I was dying! But, I had the admonition and the determination to heal myself and that's what I did!

Techniques Used:
- **Cleansing the Colon**- Rids the body of toxins and waste in order to clear the way for the healing process
- **Fresh fruits**-Cleanses and Energizes
- **Fresh Vegetables**- Builds, Tone and Heal
- **Clean Water**- Flushes and cleanses the body of toxins- life line
- **Fresh Juices**- Builds and restores the body through feeding process
- **Proper Food Combination**- Helps eliminate body dis-eases
- **Deep Air Breathing**- Strengthens the lungs, cleanses the air passages, supplies the body with oxygen ridding the body of impurities
- **Water Therapy**- (Hot water- therapy cleanses and rids the system of poisons and toxins through a sweating process) Cold water therapy- stimulates blood circulation and tones the body)
- **Turkish Towel Rub**-This technique help to stimulate the blood vessels bringing the blood to the surface to the skin, where it should flow easing discomfort and disease

- **Exercising-** Replenishes the old blood with new blood through a heating mechanism of the body-
- **Fresh Herbs-**Heals and builds and brings the body back to its natural state
- **Meditation and Visualization-** Empowers you to reach your goals

Get the Facts on
Natures Techniques to Self-Healing
And Learn the Techniques

Listen to your body. What's going on with you? Learn as much as you can about your dis-ease and then have an open mind to heal yourself.

Visualize- see yourself healed. See yourself eating good food, see yourself exercising, see yourself juicing, and see yourself going outside doing deep breathing exercises.
See yourself doing- the more you do this the stronger you will become. Keep it up don't stop!

Meditate- I_____ (your name) am now healed. I ___ (your name) am completely healthy. I love myself and I am loved. The cancer is gone or whatever illness plagues you- say it here. I am healed. I have the knowledge to be healed. I believe in myself. You may speak the desires of your heart. Just believe in yourself it will come.

First, I went out and got a juicer. If you try this you need to know not to take any fresh juice in your body until you have cleared your stomach meaning the food has passed into your colon. Then you need to clear some fecal out of your colon, so that the juice may digest easily without causing too much discomfort. It didn't take long for me to start because I was at a critical state, I just started in on my fruits and that did the job. In the morning I would get up juice apple and lemons this was one of my favorite juices

❖ *4 apples (these were organic apples)*
1 lemon

❖ *2 Pears*
2 grapefruits
1 lemon

❖ *Plain lemon water- cleanses the system*
    1 whole lemon
8oz glass of water

❖ *A good drink for cleansing*
1 lemon
Maple Syrup
Cayenne pepper
8oz glass of spring water

❖ *Citrus Boost*

2 grapefruits (peeled)
2 oranges (peeled) never do oranges if you have arthritis
1 lemon
Add a pear or apple to tone down flavor

❖ *Mango Strawberry Smoothie*
2 mangos
Cup of strawberries
2 apples- juice the apples and pour over into the blender and mixed together with the mangos and strawberries

❖ **Sweet blackberry pear juice**
½ cup of black berries
3 pears

❖ *Peach Pear Mango*
2 peaches (pitted)
2 pears
2 Mangos (pitted)

❖ *Guava Pear Juice*
3 Pears
2 guavas

    I would take a gallon of water to work with me. I drank the water in between meal time. About 30 minutes before I would have my break I wouldn't take any more water.

When break time would come I would go outside and start up my deep breathing exercises. I would take in 7 to 8 breathes through my nose hold it for just as many counts and let it out easy through my mouth. I repeated this breathing exercise 5 times. Afterwards, I would exercise mainly walking around the premises. I didn't do any strenuous exercise, because I truly found through research over exercise has an adverse effect on the body, doing more harm than good in my case getting light headed and feeling nausea. So, I exercise moderately breaking a sweat. Afterwards, I would go sit down rest a little and have my fruit.

My morning fruit (some fruits are not to mix together)
There are three varieties of fruits Sweet fruits, Acid Fruits, Sub Acid Fruits

  Sweet Fruits- Dates, Raisins, Prunes, Persimmons, Figs
    Papaya, (caution the dry fruits have additives, so make sure they're organic)

Don't Mix Sweet Fruits with Acid Fruit

Acid Fruits- Limes, Tangerines, Grapefruits, Strawberries, Oranges, Tangelos, Kiwi, Pineapple, Pomegranates, Raspberries

---

Sub-Acid Fruits- These fruits can mix with both sweet and acid fruits

Apples, Pears, Guava, Some Grapes, Cherries, Apricots, Peaches, Plums, Mangos, Nectarines   Berries – I like all my berries together – I don't like mixing them with other fruits Blackberries,

Strawberries, Blueberries, Dewberries, or any berry.

Melons alone or leave them alone

This is important- You are not to eat melons with other foods. Make sure you eat your melons by themselves. The melons ferment in your stomach with other foods when you mix them together causing discomfort (ferments meaning gas in the system) Watermelon- Honey Dew, Cantaloupe best time to eat is morning before taking in solid foods.

Reference-God Way to Ultimate Health

The more fruit you eat the faster you cleanse your body which promotes a speedy healing. Note: make sure you are combing the right fruit together to get the best benefits. I just ate until my body was satisfied. I didn't overeat, because when you overeat the waste spills over into your blood stream causing problems. Just don't overeat anything.

Back to work- keeping my water beside me. I would wait about 30 to 45 minutes before I drank more water. I only used spring water. I don't like distilled water it made me ache. So, I quick learned not to drink it. When lunch came around I ate a large green salad.

My Lunch
❖ *Romaine lettuce (Do not use iceberg lettuce)*

Mild green onions,
Cucumbers,
Organic tomatoes
Lemon freshly squeezed and poured over salad

❖ *Yellow squash Cucumber*
Purple Onions
Zucchini
Top with fresh lemon juice

❖ *Spinach (use sparingly*
Lettuce
Mild onions
Red Bell peppers

Sprinkled all salads with lemon or lime juice when cleansing

Create your own salad.............

Home for the evening. I would juice a vegetable drink.
My main drink then was carrots and apples that was back in the 90's so I have to give the credit to that drink. It help save my life. I use carrots on occasions now.

Later, I began to expound on a number of vegetables drinks. But, never mixing my vegetables and fruits together. However, apples and lemons I found seem to mix with most vegetables. In the evening I would have a plate of steam vegetables no starch at all- no potatoes, no breads etc.

My evening meals usually consisted of

❖ *Steam cabbage*
Okra
Yellow Squash
Onions

❖ *Steamed Mustard Greens*
Sautéed Onions
Green Beans
Carrots (Sometime)

❖ *red bell peppers ,yellow bell peppers, green bell peppers*
   Yellow Onions
    Garlic
Sautéed together (a big plate)

All vegetables were steamed during the cleansing phase. Once you have reached your goal, you may expound on using oil and adding little salt for taste- salt must be pure sea salt, *Note: real salt is brownish in color*. Other spices are welcome. You may use other spices during cleansing just make sure they're all fresh and pure. Myself, I only used onions and garlic.

Healing Herbs were taken after my evening dinner, I would take
I used **red clover** this was my main herb. Red clover is a great blood purifier. Today,
I mainly dig my own herbs and use them.

Water Therapy Bath (_taken before bed time_)

Water therapy rendered benefits beyond my imagination. I first ran a
tub full of hot water as hot as my body would allow. Sat a large
glass of cool water beside the tub and a large jug of ice cold water.
I got into the water and sat there until I begin to sweat. When I started
to sweat I would drank the glass of water. What happens is, the toxins
are coming out through your sweat glands and you are putting good
clean pure minerals back in your body by drinking clean water. So
whatever bad that's in the blood and muscles begins to come out than
the good stuff starts to take over. In my first stages, I did this every
day. Later, after I was feeling better I did it at least 3 times a week.
Again, once all the bad is out the good comes through your pores
rendering a transformation. When I finished with the hot bath I close
my pores with ice cold water. Pouring the water all over my body. I
would get out and finish with a technique known as a Turkish towel
rub (this is a small cotton towel- kind of rough, this technique is
needed to stimulate the cells bringing the blood to the surface of the
skin producing a glow helping to eliminate the disease. Next, I would
lay down and rest. The **rest** is highly important, making sure I wrap
myself very well before I leave the bath room, less I catch a draft. A
draft _is when air hits your wet skin and sets into your pores causing a
slight chill and you begin to sneeze as if you have a cold._ This is why
covering yourself very well is necessary. As I lay for rest my body
continued to sweat- sweating is a part of the technique as well. Your
body must be covered as you rest. Sleep follows shortly. Up the next
morning to start again. However, upon rising a tepid shower is
needed, followed by a cold shower to close your pores. Morning
showers are often taken incorrectly. We are not supposed to take a hot
shower in the morning time. Taking hot showers in the morning leaves
your pores open for unknown elements to trap themselves inside your
pores as they began to close. So, when you get up in the morning start
with a tepid shower, meaning lukewarm water, once you have finished

14

your shower close your pores with a cold shower. You will feel rejuvenated rather than tired and sluggish. I continued these techniques until I regained my health.

So roughly it took about 8 months to bring myself back to health. Now, after I did all that, I became highly fertile, I mean I was in a whole new zone. This thing was like clockwork. Healing started the latter of 1995-in October of 1996 I got pregnant and July 3, 1997 I gave birth to a beautiful little girl. Back slid slightly at no fault of my own. Then in 1998 I went into more profound study. Implementing all the techniques I had learned taking my studies to a higher level. *In*

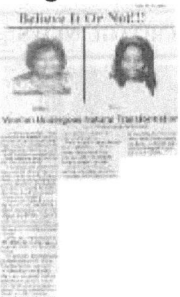

2001 I had reached unbelievable transformation. Someone said to me once, "You are determine," my reply "I guess you can say that." I have studied and researched for many years, and I want lie this thing is far from being easy. At one time on this journey from 2003-2010 I got tangled in a web of emotional, psychological upheaval that led to a physical setback. Not as ill however, some weight gain returned. This was more difficult than the first physical healing. But, again I conquered it. The experiences added to my research bringing about a stronger indebt insight of what can happen as you're on a journey to complete wellness. As you set out to conquer your hurtles, your obstacles, or whatever is holding you back, just know- no matter what it looks like, no matter how many people try to discourage you. Use their words to become stronger. Just know in your heart there is nothing that can't be done. When you get discourage read this poem

It Couldn't Be Done

BY EDGAR ALBERT GUEST

Somebody said that it couldn't be done

But he with a chuckle replied

That "maybe it couldn't," but he would be one

Who wouldn't say so till he'd tried? So he buckled right in

with the trace of a grin On his face. If he worried he hid it. He

started to sing as he tackled the thing

That couldn't be done, and he did it!

Somebody scoffed: "Oh, you'll never do that;

At least no one ever has done it;"

But he took off his coat and he took off his hat

And the first thing we knew he'd begun it.

With a lift of his chin and a bit of a grin,

Without any doubting or quiddit He started to sing as he

tackled the thing

That couldn't be done, and he did it.

There are thousands to tell you it cannot be done,

There are thousands to prophesy failure, There are thousands to

point out to you one by one,

The dangers that wait to assail you.

But just buckle in with a bit of a grin,

Just take off your coat and go to it;

Just start in to sing as you tackle the thing

That "cannot be done," and you'll do it.   I

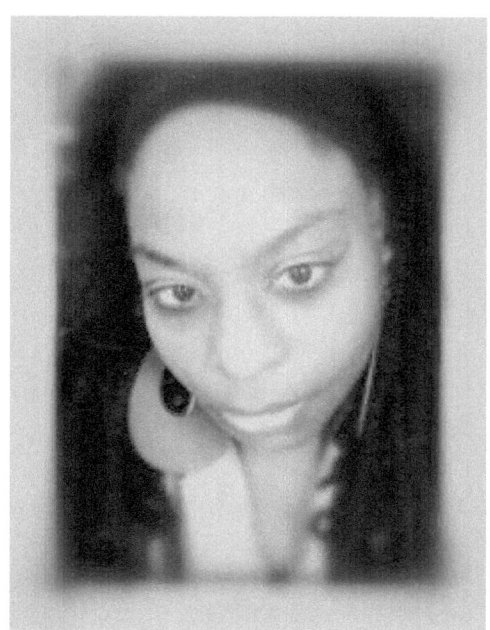

Now 14 years after the article was written.

Tips

Melons alone or leave them alone. Ever got a stomach ache after eating **watermelon.** Well that's because watermelon is made to be eating alone. It's best to take it on an empty stomach. Its' ok, the best time to eat it is morning or after you've done your exercises. You would be amazed at what it can do for you.

Did you know you are suppose too eat the entire melon. Yea! That's right! The rind and seeds too. It's made up of 90% water and highly alkaline.

The watermelon is great for the heart I know this for a fact. Juice up the rind it gets rid of pain in the joints, it is also great diuretic, and it sparks the libido. The seeds are great for food, used like sunflower seeds just eat them. However, you should stay away from seedless watermelons, my experience with seedless watermelons are poor.

Onions- did you know onions have selenium in them and they are great for asthma, the selenium put oxygen back into the lungs helping the person to breathe. Onions also have a calming effect on the body.

Jalapeno Peppers- This little pepper help me to walk. I had pulled a disk in my back years back. It hurt so bad I had to crawl on the floor, I remembered my research and that jalapeño peppers take inflammation out of the body and reduces pain. Well I juiced up a pepper took a shot, Yes I drank it straight chased it with a glass of water, instantly felt relief. In 3 days I was dancing the gig. Another thing it's good for is the kidneys it helps stimulate urine reducing the swelling and stimulating urine flow. I experienced this personally.

Cayenne Pepper- Go for the burn baby! This pepper saved my son life. He had got a hold to a food that he was highly allergic to. He heart rate was racing his breathing was irregular. I gave him about a teaspoon of cayenne in a cup of water and the child was back to normal within minutes. I was relieved to know something so simple could save a life. This pepper helps regulate the blood from head to toe.
It's nothing short of simply amazing!
You name it- it can pretty much cure it.

Mustard Greens- Anti-inflammatory, high alkaline

My opinion this is the best green in the world. Followed by Turnips greens. These are the best greens to help heal your body.

Cilantro-helps remove heavy metals from the body, powerful anti-inflammatory, helps promote healthy liver functions, helps with insulin secretion and lowers blood sugar, helps eye aging, ease conjunctivitis and muscular degeneration of the eyes.

Lemons- The best story I have to tell about lemon is it cured my little girl strep throat. Broke my children fevers and works on stopping heavy menstrual flow and aids the liver.

My Walnut Milk

I like black walnuts-the reason is I experimented with them and I know the tree. Therefore, I make my own milk from the walnuts as well eat them. Note: any highly processed walnuts are bad for you, but a good walnut will relieve pain in the body and render great nutritional benefits. (By my own research)
Take a cup or 2 of walnuts put in a blender cover with water and blend until smooth. Add some maple syrup and a little pure vanilla and there's your milk.

Pina Colada
½ Pineapple
1 can of coconut milk
Sweet to your taste
Organic Sugars are best you choose your own
Date Sugar
Maple Sugar

Maple Syrup

Honey (some wholistic doctors disagree with honey, but I have used it and experimented with it and no bad results came up. I just use it sparingly)

Green Juice

 Hand full of Mustard Greens

Jalapeño Pepper ½ or whole depends on your taste I like fire)

Green Bell pepper

For a smooth taste add a pear or apple

Great for arthritis

Nature says No To- ****Don't Eat Flesh Meat and Starches Together

Artificial meats-spam

Vienna sausages

Package sausages

Wieners

Soy patties or any soy products

Artificial chips

Sodas

Bottle juices

And sport drinks

Crackers

Candies

*Balance is needed with these items- flesh meats, pasta and breads- knowing you might not stop eating this stuff instantly unless, you are in a serious state of illness. So if you partake of these items, you **MUST Eat** them with ample amounts of **Green Vegetation**! Eat a lot of Green Stuff! And try to get **Free Range Meat** when possible.*

Powder drinks- that you add water to – anything in a package that is in a crystalize state, you need to leave it alone!

Microwaves- Kills food and the waves enter into your body each time you are close to it. Slowly having a negative effect on your body. I don't own one

Hand Sanitizers- this stuff is dangerous to the most high. 62% alcohol all alcohol % must be double to come a proof. So when you double 62% you get 124 proof. Your skin is the largest organ on your body and it leads stream and you are letting your children use it without caution. The children are becoming addicted to this stuff right in front of your faces and your eyes are close. Intoxication has been reported on several occasions. Please research this information and see for yourself.

Herbs

Mullein- this herbs is great for flu and asthma as well as getting the mucus out of your system

Sour dock- other names (yellow dock or curly dock) but when I was growing up we called it sour dock for its sour taste.
This is a blood purifier, one of the best.

Red Clover- is also a blood purifier and popular for women health

Wild Greens

Poke Salad- great wild green, good for a seasonal body cleanse. Boil the green 2x-drain and prepare Preparation varies. This green must be cooked.

Lambs quarter- This is a marvelous green, the taste Is superb and packed full of vitamins and minerals of the earth rendering what our body's needs?

Dandelion Greens- these greens grow wild and are often cut down during landscaping, however if the benefits of this green was known you would never take this little weed for granted again.

Eat plenty of Nature's Food and dis-ease will cease.

Greens Mustard
Turnips
Calilaloo
Lettuce (All types except iceberg)
Please Note: All Greens may be eaten in raw state salads can be made with any of these greens.

Bell Peppers & Peppers
Red
Green
Yellow

Jalapeno Peppers-pain reliever, and anti-inflammatory
Habanero Peppers
Cayenne Peppers

Onions
Wild green onions
Yellow onions- great for putting selenium back into lungs helping to restore free breathing
Red onions

Tomatoes-small ones cherry or plum
Tomatillo
Cucumbers-good diuretic-
Green Beans- great for diabetes
Okra- replenishes the blood- ever need a blood transfusion eat or juice okra
Squash
Olives

Spices and Seasons some may be used as tea
Thyme- reduce mucous in system
Cloves- freshens breath and aids in sore and tooth pain- also used to make clove tea
Bay leaves
Sage- healing properties
Onion Powder
Marjoram
Cumin
Ginger-used a herb tea also
 Anise - used for stomach complaints

Some things may not be mention here- don't be discourage this is only a small list of what the creator offers for good health

Thank you for reading this book. There is so much more to learn. I couldn't put everything in here, but if you ever need me to expound on this material or anything not mentioned here just contact me.   **www.ckwinsouleimane.com**

Be True to your Nature and Nature will be TRUE to you because **NATURE IS TRUE TO ALL!**

Tanya Childs-Souleimane

Reader,

I was guided by divine intervention. I read, researched and healed my body. It wasn't to years later I embarked on others that were on this same path. The information is out there if you want it.

References
Dr. Afrika-African Holistic Health
Dr. Afrika and Dr. Scott Whitaker- How to Eat to Live DVD

Dr. Sebi Products-*www.drsebiproducts.com*

Cathy Harris-The Whistle Blower

References/ Sources

A Consumer's Dictionary of Food Additives by Ruth Winter, M.S.

Back To Eden by Jethro Kloss

God's Way to Ultimate Health

"The Creator works through the Creation"

Tanya Childs-Souleimane